Welcome

Dearest Momma,

Congratulations on your tiny human! My hope is that this journal provides you the space to feel empowered throughout your pregnancy and to nurture your baby's haven during your postpartum.

Please complete the checklists as early as possible to maximize the benefits of your journal.

Hugs & Light,

Kimberly Marie

Author |Certified Doula| Certified Sleep Specialist |
Certified Breastfeeding Specialist

Prayers for My Baby

The Beginning of Forever

How I Found Out I Was Pregnant

Estimated Birth Date

Who I first told

First Ultrasound

Daily Solitude & Affirmations

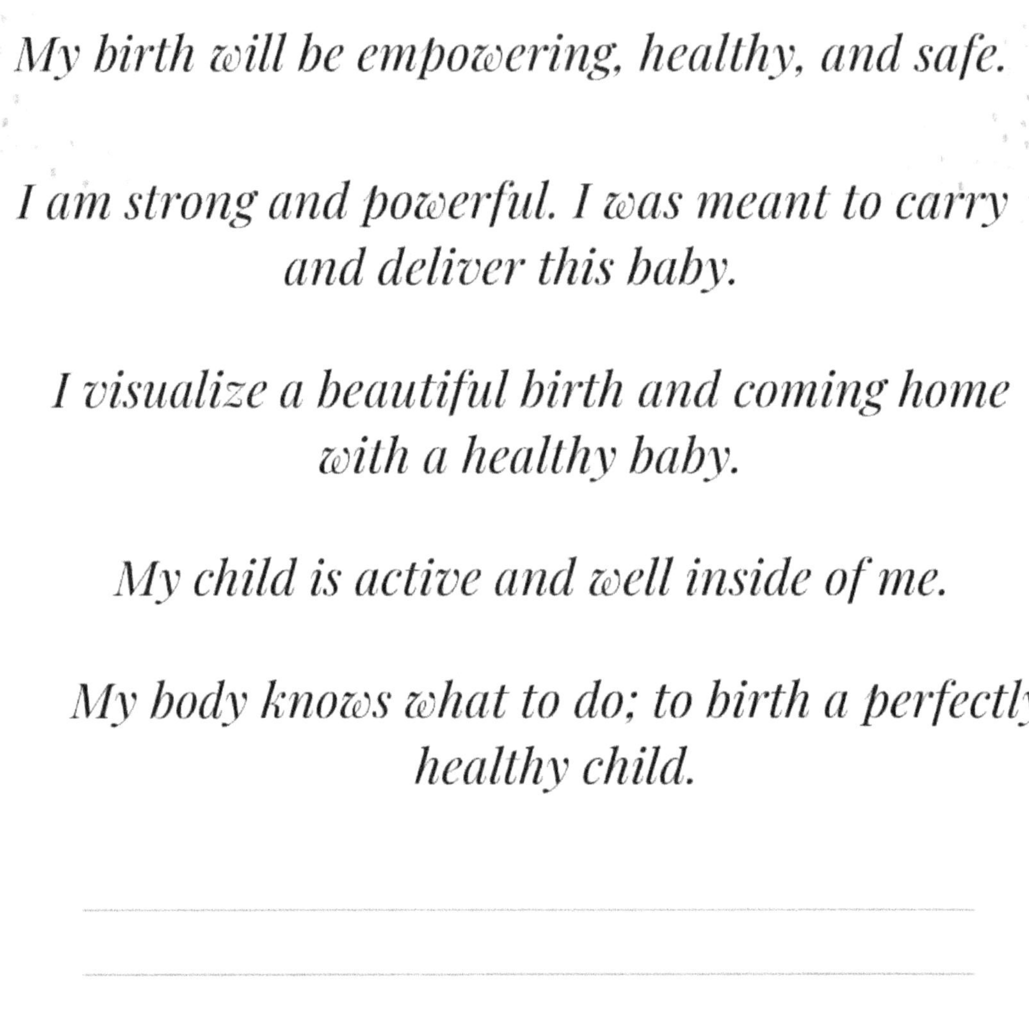

My birth will be empowering, healthy, and safe.

I am strong and powerful. I was meant to carry and deliver this baby.

I visualize a beautiful birth and coming home with a healthy baby.

My child is active and well inside of me.

My body knows what to do; to birth a perfectly healthy child.

First Trimester

First Trimester Checklist

Begin prenatal vitamin nourishment

Consider Midwifery care or OB/GYN type of prenatal care

Learn about doula care and HIRE a doula

Schedule your prenatal medical appointments

Decide on a hospital /birth center/homebirth

Switch to nourishing food and snack options

Decrease caffeine intake

Verify maternal leave allotments

Week 4
Your baby is the size of a sesame seed

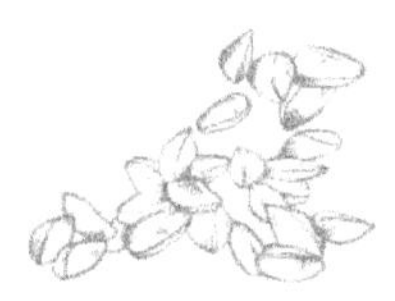

How My Body is Feeling

This Week's Challenges

Special Highlights

To-Do List

PICTURE OF MY BELLY AT 1 MONTH PREGNANT

Week 5
Your baby is The size of an orange seed

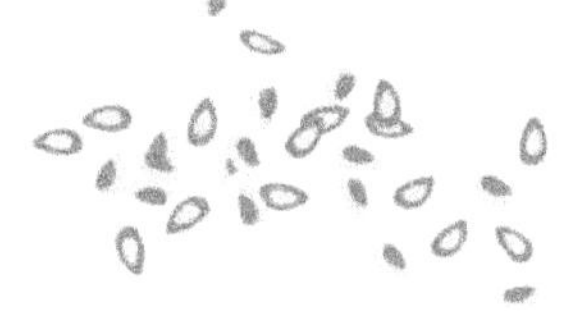

How My Body is Feeling

This Week's Challenges

Special Highlights

To-Do List

Week 6
Your baby is the size of a chocolate chip

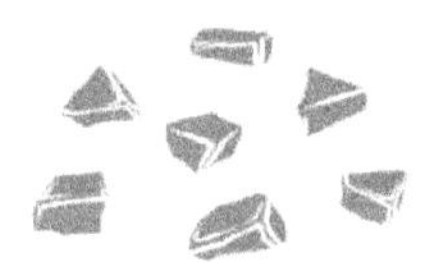

How My Body is Feeling

This Week's Challenges

Special Highlights

To-Do List

Week 7
Your baby is the size of a blueberry

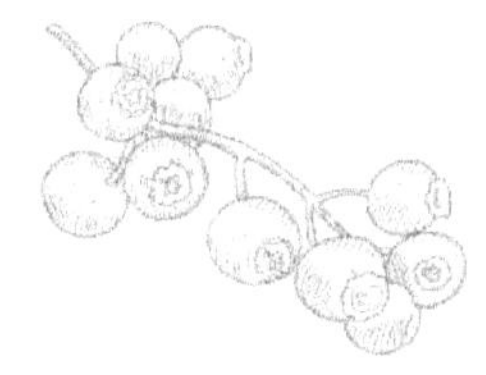

How My Body is Feeling

This Week's Challenges

Special Highlights

To-Do List

Week 8
Your baby is the size of a raspberry

How My Body is Feeling

This Week's Challenges

Special Highlights

To-Do List

PICTURE OF MY BELLY AT 2 MONTHS PREGNANT

Week 9
Your baby is the size of a grape

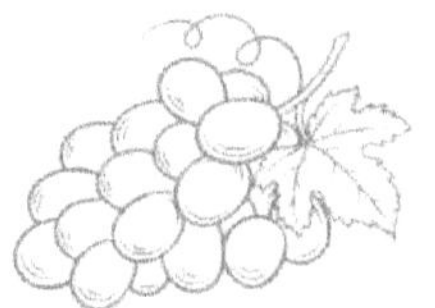

How My Body is Feeling

This Week's Challenges

Special Highlights

To-Do List

Week 10
Your baby is the size of a prune

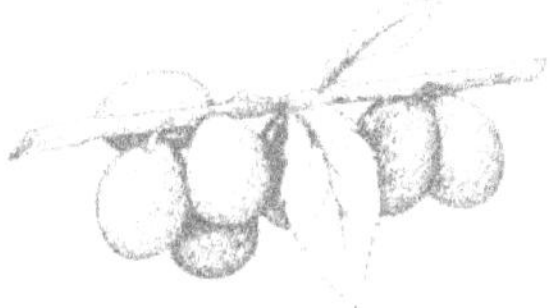

How My Body is Feeling

This Week's Challenges

Special Highlights

To-Do List

Week 11
Your baby is the size of a lime

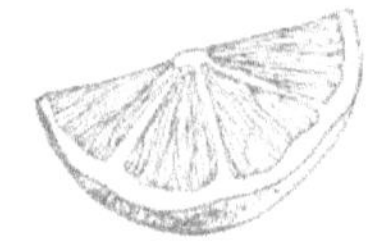

How My Body is Feeling

This Week's Challenges

Special Highlights

To-Do List

Week 12
Your baby is the size of a plum

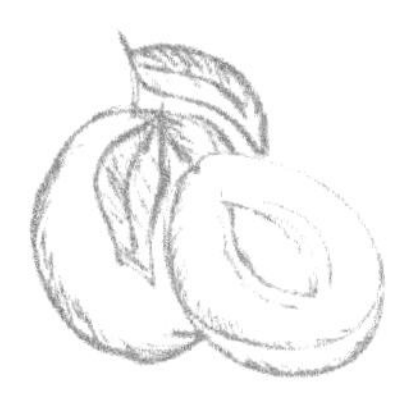

How My Body is Feeling

This Week's Challenges

Special Highlights

To-Do List

First Trimster Recap

Experiences

Emotions

Milestones

Memories

Mindful Reflections

How do I envision my birth experience

Possible Baby Names

Draw or write out how you envision your baby

Second Trimester

Second Trimester Checklist

Begin your research for Pediatrician

Create a prenatal exercise plan

Consider investing in a maternity pillow

Sign up for childbirth education classes

Plan childcare logistics

Talk to your baby

Create your baby registry

Week 13
Your baby is the size of a lemon

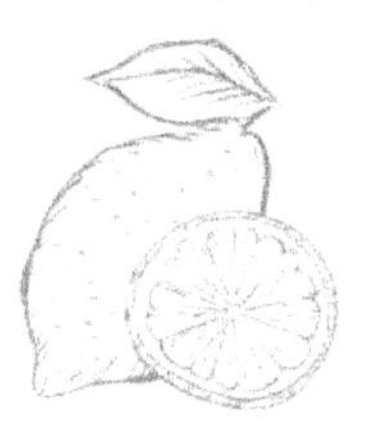

How My Body is Feeling

This Week's Challenges

Special Highlights

To-Do List

Week 14
Your baby is the size of a peach

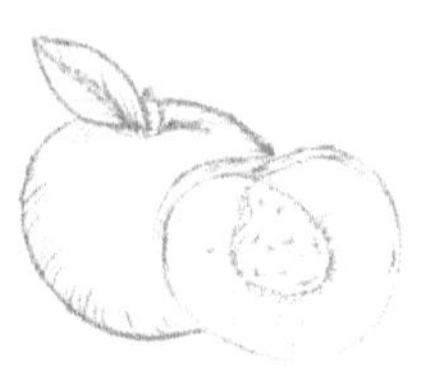

How My Body is Feeling

This Week's Challenges

Special Highlights

To-Do List

Week 15
Your baby is the size of an apple

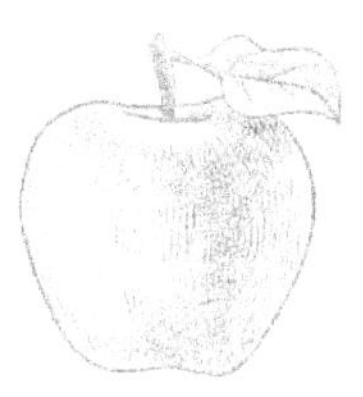

How My Body is Feeling

This Week's Challenges

Special Highlights

To-Do List

Week 16
Your baby is the size of an avocado

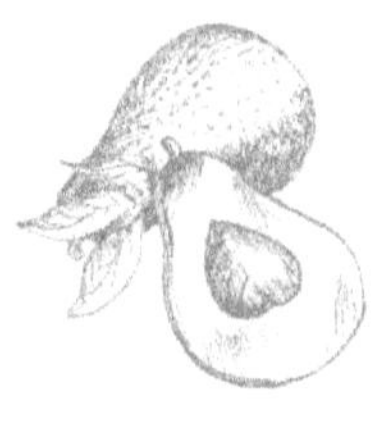

How My Body is Feeling

This Week's Challenges

Special Highlights

To-Do List

PICTURE OF MY BELLY AT 4 MONTHS PREGNANT

Week 17
Your baby is the size of a pear

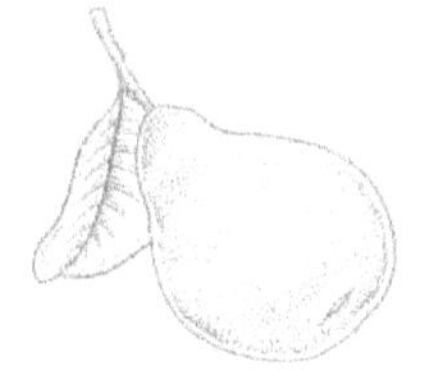

How My Body is Feeling

This Week's Challenges

Special Highlights

To-Do List

Week 18
Your baby is the size of a bell pepper

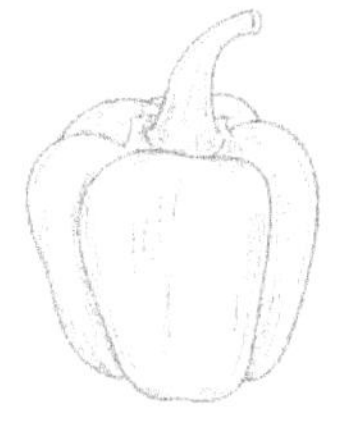

How My Body is Feeling

This Week's Challenges

Special Highlights

To-Do List

Week 19
Your baby is the size of a mango

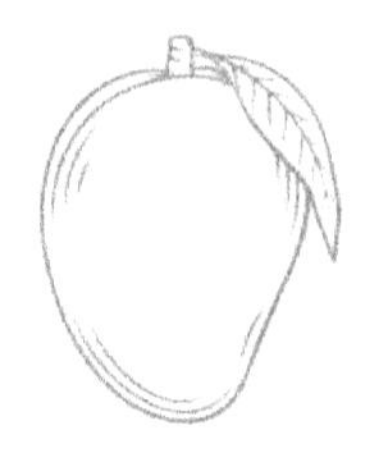

How My Body is Feeling

This Week's Challenges

Special Highlights

To-Do List

Week 20
Your baby is the size of a banana

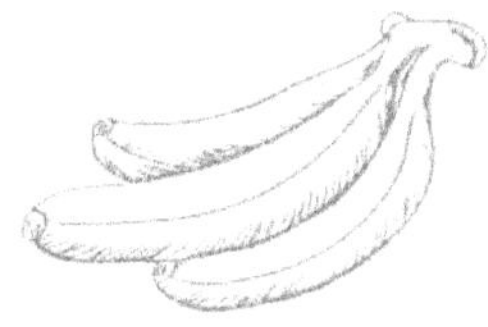

How My Body is Feeling

This Week's Challenges

Special Highlights

To-Do List

PICTURE OF MY BELLY AT 5 MONTHS PREGNANT

Week 21
Your baby is the size of a carrot

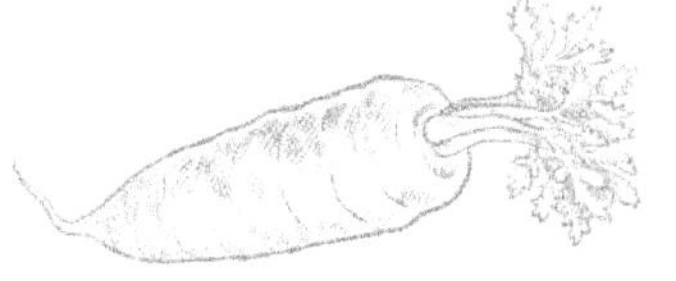

How My Body is Feeling

This Week's Challenges

Special Highlights

To-Do List

Week 22
Your baby is the size of a papaya

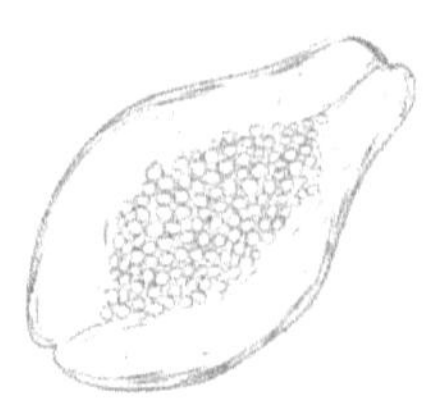

How My Body is Feeling

This Week's Challenges

Special Highlights

To-Do List

Week 23
Your baby is the size of a grapefruit

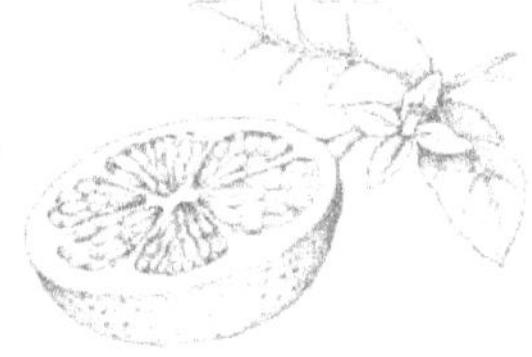

How My Body is Feeling

This Week's Challenges

Special Highlights

To-Do List

Week 24
Your baby is the size of a canteloupe

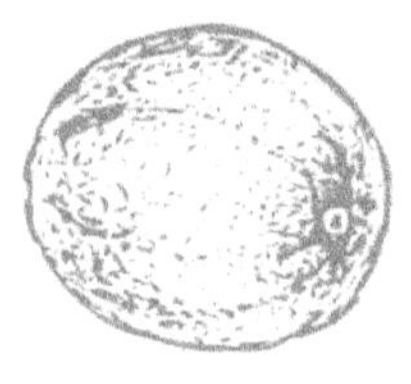

How My Body is Feeling

This Week's Challenges

Special Highlights

To-Do List

PICTURE OF MY BELLY AT 6 MONTHS PREGNANT

Week 25
Your baby is the size of a turnip

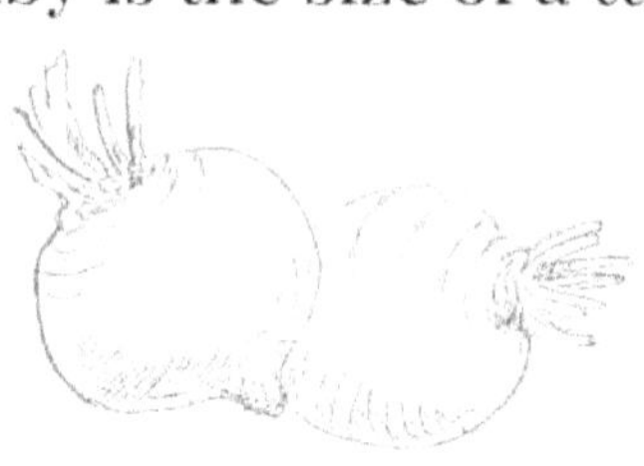

How My Body is Feeling

This Week's Challenges

Special Highlights

To-Do List

Week 26
Your baby is the size of a lettuce

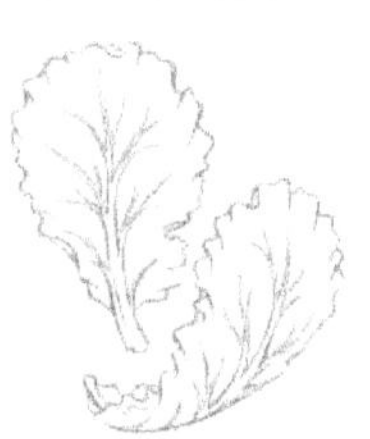

How My Body is Feeling

This Week's Challenges

Special Highlights

To-Do List

Week 27
Your baby is the size of a cauliflower

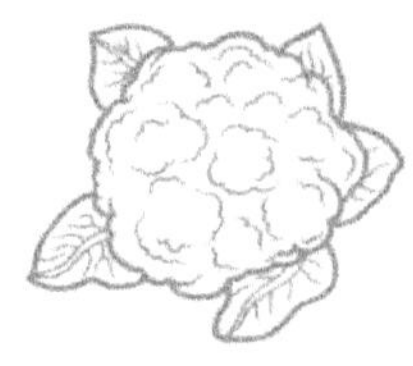

How My Body is Feeling

This Week's Challenges

Special Highlights

To-Do List

Second Trimster Recap

Experiences

Emotions

Milestones

Memories

PICTURE OF MY BELLY AT 7 MONTHS PREGNANT

Mindful Reflections

My body is incredible, this is how I practice self-love

My emotions when I first felt my baby kick

Draw or write out how you envision yourself as a parent to your baby

Third Trimester

Third Trimester Checklist

Pack your hospital bags

Download a contraction timing app

Complete the postpartum guide provided in this journal

Prioritize sleep/prayer/meditation

Wash all baby clothes

Learn about birth advocacy (provided in this journal)

Contact Vela Haven to learn about implementing
healthy sleep practices for your newborn

Week 28
Your baby is the size of an eggplant

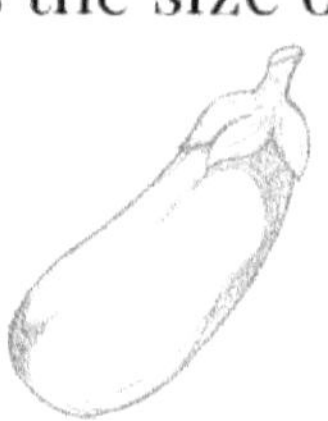

How My Body is Feeling

This Week's Challenges

Special Highlights

To-Do List

Week 29
Your baby is the size of an acorn squash

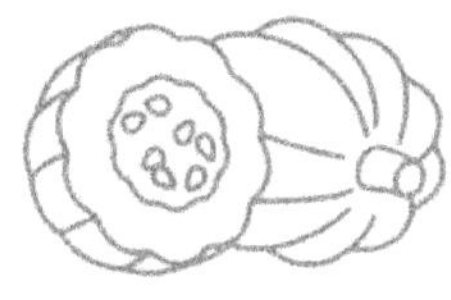

How My Body is Feeling

This Week's Challenges

Special Highlights

To-Do List

Week 30
Your baby is the size of a cabbage

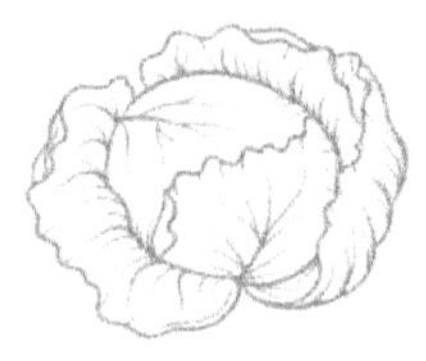

How My Body is Feeling

This Week's Challenges

Special Highlights

To-Do List

Week 31
Your baby is the size of a coconut

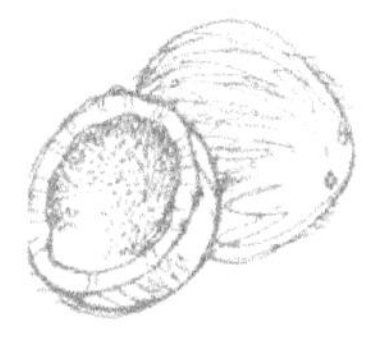

How My Body is Feeling

This Week's Challenges

Special Highlights

To-Do List

Week 32
Your baby is the size of a pineapple

How My Body is Feeling

This Week's Challenges

Special Highlights

To-Do List

PICTURE OF MY BELLY AT 8 MONTHS PREGNANT

Week 33
Your baby is the size of a butternut squash

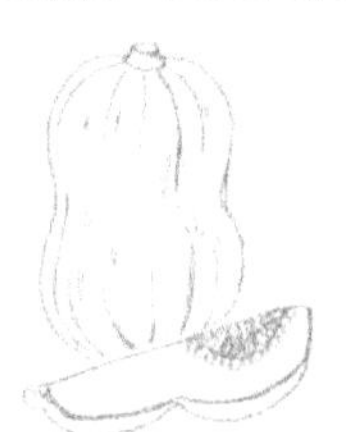

How My Body is Feeling

This Week's Challenges

Special Highlights

To-Do List

Week 34
Your baby is the size of a large canteloupe

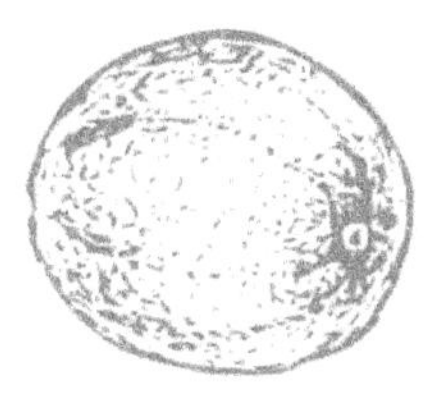

How My Body is Feeling

This Week's Challenges

Special Highlights

To-Do List

Week 35
Your baby is the size of a honeydew melon

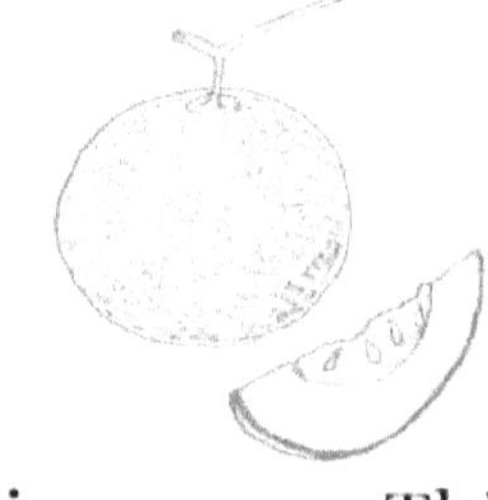

How My Body is Feeling

This Week's Challenges

Special Highlights

To-Do List

Week 36
Your baby is the size of a swiss chard

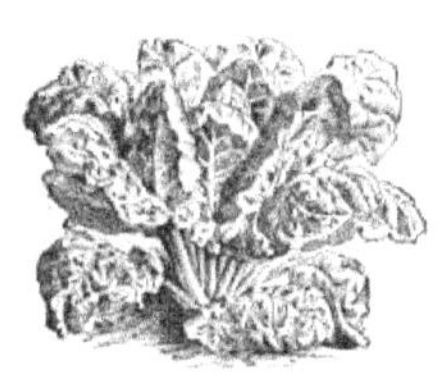

How My Body is Feeling

This Week's Challenges

Special Highlights

To-Do List

PICTURE OF MY BELLY AT 9 MONTHS PREGNANT

Week 37
Your baby is the size of a winter melon

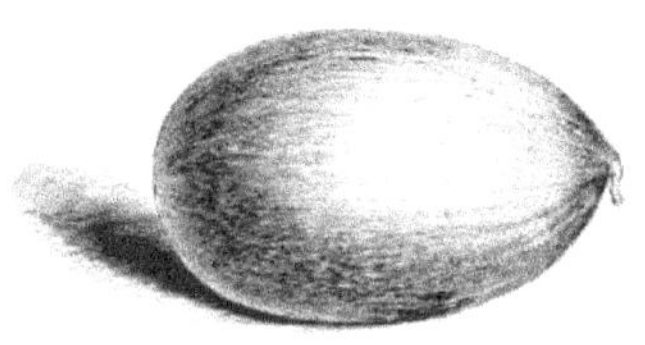

How My Body is Feeling

This Week's Challenges

Special Highlights

To-Do List

Week 38
Your baby is the size of a rhubarb

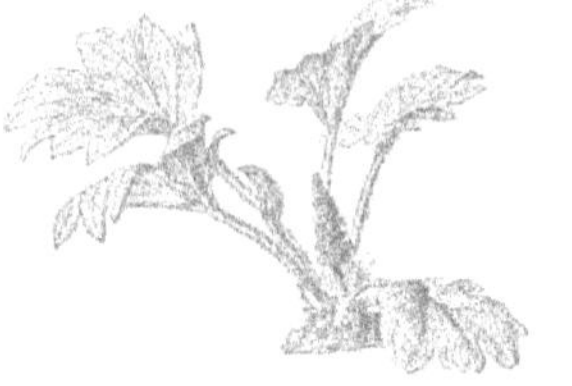

How My Body is Feeling

This Week's Challenges

Special Highlights

To-Do List

Week 39
Your baby is the size of a pumpkin

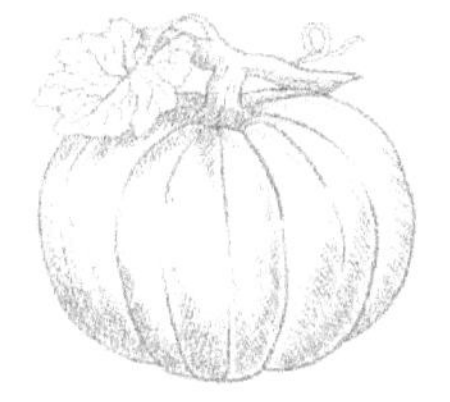

How My Body is Feeling

This Week's Challenges

Special Highlights

To-Do List

Week 40
Your baby is the size of a large jackfruit

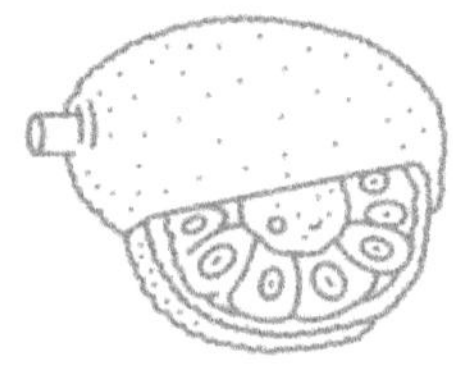

How My Body is Feeling

This Week's Challenges

Special Highlights

To-Do List

Third Trimster Recap

Experiences

Emotions

Milestones

Memories

PICTURE OF MY BELLY AT 10 MONTHS PREGNANT

Week 41

How My Body is Feeling

This Week's Challenges

Special Highlights

To-Do List

Week 42

How My Body is Feeling

This Week's Challenges

Special Highlights

To-Do List

Postpartum Preparation

Postpartum Planning Activity

What are your worries about postpartum changes?

What are your fears about motherhood?

Who will be your hands-on support throughout the first 6 weeks of your recovery?

Meal Preparation & Planning

Mommy Happiness List- Postpartum Guide

Please ensure the guide below is presented to your partner, family members, or any person who will assist you throughout your postpartum journey

If I am overwhelmed, please offer to help me in this way:

My postpartum period is sacred. Please, no visitors at these times:

Surprise me with some of my favorite things or comfort foods such as:

I would appreciate if you would take initiative and clean up these areas:

Postpartum depression is very real. If you notice I am not myself in any extreme or unusual way, please call my:

Therapist:

Doctor:

Doula:

Sometimes I may cry, stress-out, be sad, or overwhelmed and I may not say it. PLEASE FREQUENTLY ASK ME "HOW I AM DOING/HOW CAN I HELP"

Postpartum Healing Checklist

Hire Post Partum Doula

Research perinatal mood disorders

'At home' blood pressure machine

Key phone numbers: therapist, practitioners, doula

Verify/ confirm maternal leave from work

Post partum pads/diapers

Peri bottles (1 for each restroom)

Ice pack

Warm compress

Healing womb tea

Herbal healing bath

Sitz bath

Confirm post partum plans with family

Questions for my pregnancy care provider

What are my birthing options?

What is a healthy amount of weight gain throughout pregnancy?

Recommendations to aid with physical discomfort?

What foods or physical activities should I avoid?

Who are your back up practitioners/midwives?

Do you routinely use interventions at birth?

Can we review my birth preferences?

Is my doula allowed to support me at birth?

Are you open to working with my doula as a part of my birth team?

Labor Advocacy Preparation

This intervention isn't apart of my birth preference. How is it advantageous to me?

What does evidence based research show about this option?

Are there any risks?

Are my baby and I ok?

Will this option cause my baby to be in distress?

Do you routinely use interventions at birth?

As long as I am fine and my baby is ok, I would prefer to avoid any unnecessary interferences at my birth

Birthing Bag Essentials-For Hospital & Home Births

Birth Preferences

Comfortable Clothing

Snacks and more snacks

Comfort Tools

Insurance Documents

Birthing Playlists

Hair Bands

Lip Chapstick

Essential Oils

Toiletries

Tools to make your birthing space comfortable

Fuzzy socks

Maternity Underwear

Pajama Nightwear

Pillows, Ice Chips & Popsiles

Water Bottle with straw

Extension Cable

Phone Charger

Anything you need to create a peaceful & empowering birth environment

Birthing Bag Essentials–For Baby

Carseat properly installed in your car

Car Seat Cover

New Born Diapers

Unscented Wipes

Receiving Blankets

Comfy Blankets

Socks

Hats

Booties

Mittens

Onesies

Pajamas

First Picture Outfit

Going Home Outfit

Nursing Pillow

My Baby's Birth Story

First Baby's Photo After Birth

Dedication to my Baby

This journal has been a labor of love for me, and it is intended to help make pregnancy and childbirth safe and comfortable. While you cannot prepare for every possibility, knowing that you are as equipped as possible promotes a calm and healthy experience. Each activity and checklist are intended to provide guidance and you should add your own must haves and questions to personalize it and make it yours. Record the great moments, the growth, and even the rough times so you can reflect on them later and provide your child with a look into your personal experience during this time.

Please use each of the pages to track your weekly progress and prepare your family for the upcoming experiences. Each checklist can be printed and kept in an easy to see place as you finish each task. The included encouragement for family and friends can be copied and given to your support team and loved ones to help you feel empowered and assisted. These tools have been created for you to use and reuse as needed. Complete each section as you progress and add in your own notes and stories as you see fit. This journal is meant to later remind you of such a cherished time in your life, and to work through the planning and emotions that come along with it.

Thank you for allowing me to be a part of your journey in this way.

With Love,

Kim